DR. BARBARA'S 7 DAYS HERBAL SMOOTHIES DETOX

Ultimate guide to approved natural and holistic approaches to full-body detox, kidney, liver and lungs cleanse for optimal wellness

Ben Hans

Table of Contents

COPYRIGHT © 2023

CHAPTER ONE

Introduction to Smoothies Detox: Understanding Its Benefits

Smoothie detox has emerged as a popular trend in the realm of health and wellness, promising a plethora of benefits ranging from weight loss to improved digestion and increased energy levels. This comprehensive guide aims to delve into the intricacies of smoothie detox, shedding light on its benefits, mechanisms, and practical implementation.

Understanding Detoxification:

Detoxification is the process through which the body eliminates toxins and waste products, ensuring optimal functioning of organs and systems. While the human body possesses its own detoxification mechanisms primarily through the liver, kidneys, and skin, external factors such as poor dietary choices, environmental pollutants, and stress can overload these natural processes, leading to a buildup of toxins. This accumulation can manifest as fatigue, digestive issues, skin problems, and more.

Smoothie Detox: A Holistic Approach:

Smoothie detox entails the consumption of nutrient-rich beverages made from fresh fruits, vegetables, and other healthful ingredients to support the body's detoxification processes. Unlike traditional juice cleanses, which often lack fiber and essential nutrients, smoothie detox offers a more balanced approach by retaining the fiber content of fruits and vegetables, promoting satiety and stable blood sugar levels.

Benefits of Smoothie Detox:

1. **Nutrient-Rich:** Smoothie detox provides a concentrated dose of vitamins, minerals, antioxidants, and phytonutrients essential for cellular repair and regeneration. By incorporating a variety of fruits and vegetables into smoothies, individuals can ensure adequate intake of micronutrients crucial for overall health and well-being.

2. **Hydration:** Many fruits and vegetables boast high water content, contributing to hydration levels in the body. Proper hydration is vital for optimal organ function, toxin elimination, and metabolic processes. Smoothie detox offers a delicious and convenient way to boost fluid intake, especially for individuals who struggle to meet their daily water requirements.

3. **Digestive Health:** The fiber present in fruits and vegetables supports digestive health by promoting regular bowel movements, preventing constipation, and supporting the growth of beneficial gut bacteria. Smoothie detox can aid in alleviating digestive discomfort and improving overall gut function, leading to enhanced nutrient absorption and waste elimination.

4. **Weight Management:** Incorporating smoothie detox into a balanced diet can facilitate weight management efforts. By replacing calorie-dense and processed foods with nutrient-dense smoothies, individuals may experience reduced calorie intake while still satisfying their hunger and nutritional needs. Additionally, the fiber content of smoothies promotes feelings of fullness, reducing the likelihood of overeating.

5. **Increased Energy Levels:** Consuming a diet rich in fruits, vegetables, and whole foods provides the body with sustained energy throughout the day. Smoothie detox can help stabilize blood sugar levels, preventing energy crashes associated with consumption of refined sugars and processed foods. The vitamins and minerals present in smoothies also support mitochondrial function, the powerhouse of cells responsible for energy production.

6. **Enhanced Detoxification:** Certain ingredients commonly used in smoothie detox recipes, such as leafy greens, citrus fruits, and cruciferous vegetables, contain compounds that support the body's natural detoxification pathways. These include antioxidants like vitamin C, glutathione, and phytochemicals, which help neutralize free radicals and facilitate the elimination of toxins from the body.

7. **Improved Skin Health:** The abundance of vitamins, minerals, and antioxidants in smoothie detox can contribute to improved skin health and complexion. Nutrients like vitamin E, vitamin C, and beta-carotene promote collagen production, reduce inflammation, and protect against oxidative stress, leading to clearer, more radiant skin.

Conclusion:

Smoothie detox offers a holistic approach to supporting the body's natural detoxification processes while providing an array of health benefits. By incorporating nutrient-rich ingredients into delicious and convenient beverages, individuals can enhance their overall well-being, promote weight management, and boost energy levels. However, it's essential to complement smoothie detox with a balanced diet and lifestyle practices to maximize its effectiveness and ensure long-term health and vitality.

CHAPTER TWO

Meet Dr. Barbara: Her Background and Expertise in Herbal Medicine

Dr. Barbara is a renowned herbalist with a wealth of knowledge and experience in the field of alternative medicine. Her journey into herbal medicine began with a deep-rooted passion for plants and their therapeutic properties, which she cultivated from a young age. This comprehensive exploration will delve into Dr. Barbara's background, her expertise in herbal medicine, and the invaluable contributions she has made to the field.

Early Influences and Education:

Dr. Barbara's fascination with plants and their healing properties was sparked during her childhood spent in the countryside, where she developed a profound appreciation for nature's bounty. Growing up surrounded by lush forests, fragrant gardens, and medicinal herbs, she felt a deep connection to the natural world and harbored a curiosity about the potential of plants to promote health and wellness.

Her academic journey began with a degree in botany, where she immersed herself in the study of plant biology, ecology, and pharmacognosy—the branch of pharmacology concerned with the discovery and study of natural products from plants. This foundational knowledge laid the groundwork for her subsequent foray into herbal medicine, providing her with a solid understanding of plant anatomy, biochemistry, and pharmacology.

Professional Development and Specialization:

Following her undergraduate studies, Dr. Barbara pursued advanced training in herbal medicine, seeking out mentors and experts in the field to expand her knowledge and hone her skills. She embarked on a journey of discovery, delving into ancient healing traditions, indigenous knowledge systems, and modern scientific research to deepen her understanding of herbal remedies and their therapeutic applications.

Dr. Barbara's approach to herbal medicine is holistic and integrative, drawing inspiration from diverse healing modalities, including Traditional Chinese Medicine, Ayurveda, Western herbalism, and indigenous plant medicine practices. She recognizes the importance of honoring traditional wisdom while integrating evidence-based research and clinical experience to inform her practice.

Throughout her career, Dr. Barbara has focused on developing a comprehensive understanding of medicinal plants, their active constituents, and their mechanisms of action within the body. She has conducted extensive research into the pharmacological properties of herbs, exploring their potential therapeutic effects on various health conditions, from chronic inflammation and immune disorders to digestive disturbances and stress-related ailments.

Contributions to the Field:

Dr. Barbara's expertise in herbal medicine has led to numerous contributions to the field, including educational initiatives, public outreach programs, and professional collaborations. She is passionate about sharing her knowledge and empowering individuals to take control of their health through natural means.

As a respected educator, Dr. Barbara has taught courses and workshops on herbal medicine, botanical identification, and holistic wellness, inspiring countless students to explore the healing potential of plants. She has also authored articles, books, and research papers, disseminating valuable information about herbal remedies and their applications in clinical practice.

In addition to her educational endeavors, Dr. Barbara is actively involved in community outreach and advocacy efforts to promote access to herbal medicine and support sustainable practices. She advocates for the preservation of medicinal plant ecosystems, ethical harvesting practices, and the cultivation of medicinal herbs to ensure their availability for future generations.

Conclusion:

Dr. Barbara's background and expertise in herbal medicine reflect a lifelong commitment to exploring the healing power of plants and sharing her knowledge with others. Through her dedication to education, research, and advocacy, she has made significant contributions to the field of alternative medicine, inspiring individuals to embrace natural approaches to health and wellness. Her holistic perspective, grounded in both tradition and science, serves as a guiding light for those seeking to harness the therapeutic potential of medicinal plants for optimal health and vitality.

CHAPTER THREE

The Science Behind Smoothie Detox: How They Support Cleansing and Health

Smoothie detox has gained popularity as a method for supporting the body's natural cleansing processes and promoting overall health and well-being. While the concept of detoxification has been a cornerstone of traditional healing practices for centuries, the science behind smoothie detox lies in understanding how specific nutrients and ingredients in these beverages support the body's detoxification pathways. This exploration will delve into the scientific principles underlying smoothie detox and elucidate how these nutrient-rich beverages can facilitate cleansing and promote optimal health.

Nutrient Density and Bioavailability:

One of the key principles of smoothie detox is the emphasis on nutrient density—the concentration of vitamins, minerals, antioxidants, and phytonutrients in the ingredients used to prepare the smoothie. Fruits and vegetables, the primary components of smoothies, are rich sources of essential nutrients that play critical roles in supporting detoxification pathways.

The bioavailability of nutrients in smoothies is enhanced through the blending process, which breaks down cell walls and releases nutrients from plant cells, making them more readily absorbable by the body. This increased bioavailability ensures that the body can efficiently utilize the nutrients present in smoothies to support detoxification processes and promote overall health.

Antioxidant Support:

Many fruits and vegetables used in smoothie detox are rich in antioxidants, compounds that help neutralize free radicals and protect cells from oxidative damage. Oxidative stress, caused by an imbalance between free radicals and antioxidants in the body, can contribute to inflammation, cellular damage, and chronic disease.

By incorporating antioxidant-rich ingredients such as berries, leafy greens, and citrus fruits into smoothies, individuals can provide their bodies with ample antioxidant support, helping to combat oxidative stress and promote cellular health. Antioxidants also play a crucial role in supporting liver function, the primary organ responsible for detoxification, by aiding in the breakdown and elimination of toxins from the body.

Fiber and Digestive Health:

Fiber is another essential component of smoothie detox that supports the body's natural cleansing processes. Fruits and vegetables are excellent sources of dietary fiber, which plays a vital role in promoting digestive health and regularity. Fiber acts as a bulking agent in the digestive tract, helping to absorb water and facilitate the movement of waste through the intestines.

The fiber content of smoothies helps promote satiety, regulate blood sugar levels, and support the growth of beneficial gut bacteria. A healthy gut microbiome is essential for proper digestion, nutrient absorption, and toxin elimination. By incorporating fiber-rich ingredients such as spinach, kale, and flaxseeds into smoothies, individuals can support optimal digestive function and promote overall detoxification.

Hydration and Fluid Balance:

Proper hydration is essential for supporting detoxification processes, as water plays a crucial role in flushing toxins from the body via urine, sweat, and respiration. Many fruits and vegetables used in smoothie detox have high water content, contributing to hydration levels and supporting fluid balance.

Incorporating hydrating ingredients such as cucumber, celery, and watermelon into smoothies can help individuals maintain optimal hydration levels, ensuring efficient detoxification and promoting overall health and well-being.

Conclusion:

The science behind smoothie detox revolves around understanding how nutrient-rich ingredients support the body's natural cleansing processes and promote optimal health. By incorporating antioxidant-rich fruits and vegetables, fiber, hydration, and other healthful ingredients into smoothies, individuals can provide their bodies with the essential nutrients and hydration needed to support detoxification pathways. Smoothie detox offers a convenient and delicious way to support overall health and well-being while promoting cellular health, digestive function, and toxin elimination.

CHAPTER FOUR

Getting Started: Preparing Mentally and Physically for the Detox

Embarking on a smoothie detox journey requires careful preparation, both mentally and physically, to set oneself up for success and maximize the benefits of the cleanse. This section will explore essential steps to take before starting a detox, focusing on mental readiness, dietary adjustments, and lifestyle modifications necessary to support the body during the cleansing process.

Mental Preparation:

1. **Set Clear Intentions:** Before beginning a detox, it's essential to clarify your reasons for undertaking the cleanse and establish clear goals. Whether you're looking to boost energy levels, jumpstart weight loss, or support overall health, articulating your intentions will help you stay motivated and committed throughout the process.

2. **Cultivate a Positive Mindset:** Approach the detox with a positive mindset, focusing on the benefits it will bring rather than viewing it as a restrictive or daunting experience. Embrace the opportunity for renewal and rejuvenation, and remind yourself of the positive changes you're making to support your health and well-being.

3. **Practice Mindfulness:** Cultivate mindfulness and self-awareness throughout the detox process, paying attention to your thoughts, feelings, and bodily sensations. Take time for reflection and introspection, noticing any patterns or habits that may be hindering your health goals and identifying areas for growth and improvement.

Physical Preparation:

1. **Gradual Dietary Adjustments:** Ease into the detox process by gradually eliminating processed foods, refined sugars, caffeine, and alcohol from your diet in the days leading up to the cleanse. This gradual transition will help reduce withdrawal symptoms and minimize potential detox reactions.

2. **Hydration:** Prioritize hydration by increasing your water intake in the days leading up to the detox. Proper hydration is essential for supporting detoxification processes, flushing toxins from the body, and maintaining optimal cellular function. Aim to drink at least eight glasses of water per day, and consider incorporating hydrating foods such as cucumber, watermelon, and citrus fruits into your diet.

3. **Stock Up on Supplies:** Ensure you have all the necessary ingredients and supplies on hand before starting the detox. Stock up on a variety of fresh fruits, vegetables, leafy greens, herbs, and other ingredients needed to prepare nutrient-rich

smoothies. Invest in a high-quality blender or juicer to facilitate the smoothie-making process and ensure smooth, creamy blends.

4. **Meal Planning:** Plan your meals and snacks ahead of time to ensure you have nutritious options available throughout the detox. Incorporate a balance of fruits, vegetables, whole grains, lean proteins, and healthy fats into your meals to provide essential nutrients and support energy levels.

5. **Sleep and Rest:** Prioritize sleep and restorative practices to support your body's natural detoxification processes. Aim for seven to nine hours of quality sleep per night, and incorporate relaxation techniques such as meditation, deep breathing, and gentle stretching into your daily routine to promote relaxation and stress relief.

Conclusion:

Preparing mentally and physically for a smoothie detox is essential for setting the stage for a successful cleanse and maximizing the benefits of the experience. By cultivating a positive mindset, making gradual dietary adjustments, prioritizing hydration, stocking up on supplies, planning meals, and prioritizing sleep and rest, you can lay the foundation for a transformative detox journey that supports your health and well-being. Remember to approach the detox with patience, self-

compassion, and a willingness to embrace the process of renewal
and rejuvenation.

CHAPTER FIVE

Essential Ingredients: Exploring Detoxifying Herbs, Fruits, and Vegetables

Detoxifying smoothies rely on a diverse array of herbs, fruits, and vegetables packed with vitamins, minerals, antioxidants, and phytonutrients to support the body's natural cleansing processes. This section will delve into some of the essential ingredients commonly used in detox smoothies, highlighting their detoxifying properties and health benefits.

1. Leafy Greens:

Leafy greens such as spinach, kale, Swiss chard, and collard greens are nutritional powerhouses rich in chlorophyll, antioxidants, and fiber. Chlorophyll, the pigment responsible for the green color of plants, has been shown to support liver detoxification by binding to toxins and promoting their elimination from the body. Additionally, leafy greens are excellent sources of vitamins A, C, and K, as well as minerals such as iron and magnesium, which support overall health and vitality.

2. Citrus Fruits:

Citrus fruits like lemons, limes, oranges, and grapefruits are prized for their high vitamin C content and alkalizing properties. Vitamin C is a potent antioxidant that supports immune function, collagen synthesis, and detoxification processes in the body.

Citrus fruits also contain flavonoids and limonoids, compounds that have been shown to support liver health and aid in the elimination of toxins.

3. Berries:

Berries such as strawberries, blueberries, raspberries, and blackberries are antioxidant-rich fruits that boast a wide range of health benefits. These vibrant fruits are packed with anthocyanins, flavonoids, and other phytochemicals that help combat oxidative stress, inflammation, and cellular damage. Berries also contain fiber, which supports digestive health and promotes satiety, making them an excellent addition to detox smoothies.

4. Cruciferous Vegetables:

Cruciferous vegetables like broccoli, cauliflower, Brussels sprouts, and cabbage are renowned for their detoxifying properties and unique sulfur-containing compounds known as glucosinolates. These compounds have been shown to support liver detoxification pathways, enhance antioxidant activity, and reduce the risk of chronic diseases such as cancer. Incorporating cruciferous vegetables into detox smoothies can help promote overall health and well-being.

5. Herbs and Spices:

Herbs and spices such as ginger, turmeric, cilantro, parsley, and mint are valued for their potent detoxifying and anti-inflammatory properties. Ginger and turmeric, in particular, contain bioactive compounds like gingerol and curcumin, which have been shown to support digestion, reduce inflammation, and enhance detoxification processes. Fresh herbs like cilantro and parsley are also believed to aid in heavy metal detoxification by binding to toxins and facilitating their removal from the body.

6. Detoxifying Teas:

Herbal teas such as dandelion root tea, green tea, and nettle tea are popular additions to detox smoothies due to their cleansing and diuretic properties. Dandelion root tea, in particular, is prized for its ability to support liver function, promote bile production, and aid in the elimination of toxins from the body. Green tea contains catechins, antioxidants that have been shown to support metabolism and enhance detoxification processes.

Conclusion:

Incorporating a variety of detoxifying herbs, fruits, and vegetables into smoothies can provide the body with essential nutrients, antioxidants, and phytonutrients to support its natural cleansing processes. From leafy greens and citrus fruits to berries, cruciferous vegetables, herbs, and detoxifying teas, these ingredients offer a potent blend of health-promoting properties that can help rejuvenate and revitalize the body from the inside out. Experiment with different combinations and flavors to create delicious and nourishing smoothies that support your health and well-being.

CHAPTER SIX

Day 1: Cleansing Green Smoothies for Energy Boost

Embarking on a smoothie detox journey begins with a focus on energizing green smoothies packed with nutrient-rich ingredients to kickstart your day on a vibrant note. These cleansing green smoothies are designed to provide a burst of energy, support detoxification processes, and nourish your body with essential vitamins, minerals, and antioxidants. Below are three refreshing green smoothie recipes to fuel your Day 1 of the detox:

1. Green Goddess Smoothie:

Ingredients:

- 1 cup spinach leaves

- 1/2 cup cucumber, chopped

- 1/2 green apple, cored and chopped

- 1/4 avocado, peeled and pitted

- 1 tablespoon fresh lemon juice

- 1 teaspoon grated ginger

- 1 cup coconut water or almond milk

- Ice cubes (optional)

Instructions:

1. Place all the ingredients in a blender.

2. Blend until smooth and creamy, adding more liquid if necessary to reach your desired consistency.

3. Pour into glasses and enjoy immediately.

2. Detoxifying Green Citrus Smoothie:

Ingredients:

- 1 cup kale leaves, stems removed

- 1/2 cup pineapple chunks

- 1/2 orange, peeled and segmented

- 1/2 lime, juiced

- 1 tablespoon fresh mint leaves

- 1 tablespoon chia seeds

- 1 cup coconut water or water

- Ice cubes (optional)

Instructions:

1. In a blender, combine the kale, pineapple, orange segments, lime juice, mint leaves, chia seeds, and coconut water.

2. Blend until smooth and creamy, adjusting the consistency with more liquid if needed.

3. Serve immediately with ice cubes if desired.

3. Energizing Green Banana Smoothie:

Ingredients:

- 1 cup spinach or kale leaves

- 1 ripe banana, peeled

- 1/2 cup sliced cucumber

- 1/4 cup fresh parsley leaves

- 1 tablespoon almond butter or peanut butter

- 1 tablespoon hemp seeds

- 1 teaspoon honey or maple syrup (optional)

- 1 cup unsweetened almond milk or coconut water

- Ice cubes (optional)

Instructions:

1. Place the spinach or kale, banana, cucumber, parsley leaves, almond butter, hemp seeds, honey or maple syrup (if using), and almond milk or coconut water in a blender.

2. Blend until smooth and creamy, adding more liquid if necessary.

3. Pour into glasses, add ice cubes if desired, and enjoy immediately.

Conclusion:

These cleansing green smoothies are perfect for Day 1 of your detox journey, providing a refreshing and nourishing way to kickstart your day with energy and vitality. Packed with nutrient-rich ingredients like leafy greens, fruits, herbs, and seeds, these smoothies offer a delicious and convenient way to support detoxification processes while fueling your body with essential nutrients. Experiment with different combinations and flavors to find your favorite green smoothie recipes and enjoy the benefits of vibrant health and energy throughout your detox journey.

CHAPTER SEVEN

Day 2-6: Daily Smoothie Recipes for Detoxification and Nutrient Replenishment

As you continue your smoothie detox journey, it's essential to vary your daily smoothie recipes to ensure you're receiving a diverse array of nutrients while supporting your body's detoxification processes. Below are five daily smoothie recipes designed to promote detoxification, replenish nutrients, and keep you feeling energized and revitalized throughout Days 2-6 of your detox:

Day 2: Berry Detox Blast

Ingredients:

- 1 cup mixed berries (such as strawberries, blueberries, raspberries)
- 1/2 cup spinach leaves
- 1/2 ripe banana
- 1 tablespoon chia seeds
- 1 tablespoon fresh lemon juice
- 1 cup coconut water or almond milk
- Ice cubes (optional)

Instructions:

1. Combine all ingredients in a blender.

2. Blend until smooth and creamy.

3. Pour into glasses and serve immediately.

Day 3: Tropical Green Refresher

Ingredients:

- 1/2 cup pineapple chunks
- 1/2 cup mango chunks
- 1 cup spinach or kale leaves
- 1/4 avocado, peeled and pitted
- 1 tablespoon fresh lime juice
- 1 tablespoon coconut flakes
- 1 cup coconut water or water
- Ice cubes (optional)

Instructions:

1. Place all ingredients in a blender.

2. Blend until smooth and creamy.

3. Pour into glasses and enjoy immediately.

Day 4: Citrus Green Detox

Ingredients:

- 1/2 grapefruit, peeled and segmented
- 1/2 orange, peeled and segmented
- 1 cup spinach or kale leaves
- 1/2 cucumber, chopped
- 1 tablespoon fresh mint leaves
- 1 tablespoon hemp seeds
- 1 cup coconut water or water
- Ice cubes (optional)

Instructions:

1. Add all ingredients to a blender.
2. Blend until smooth and creamy.
3. Pour into glasses and serve immediately.

Day 5: Creamy Green Protein Smoothie

Ingredients:

- 1/2 cup Greek yogurt or plant-based yogurt
- 1/2 ripe avocado, peeled and pitted

- 1/2 cup spinach or kale leaves

- 1/2 cucumber, chopped

- 1 tablespoon almond butter or peanut butter

- 1 tablespoon hemp seeds

- 1 teaspoon honey or maple syrup (optional)

- 1 cup almond milk or coconut water

- Ice cubes (optional)

Instructions:

1. Combine all ingredients in a blender.

2. Blend until smooth and creamy.

3. Pour into glasses and enjoy immediately.

Day 6: Green Superfood Elixir

Ingredients:

- 1 cup spinach or kale leaves

- 1/2 cucumber, chopped

- 1/2 green apple, cored and chopped

- 1 tablespoon fresh parsley leaves

- 1 tablespoon fresh ginger, grated

- 1 tablespoon chia seeds

- Juice of 1 lemon

- 1 cup coconut water or water

- Ice cubes (optional)

Instructions:

1. Place all ingredients in a blender.

2. Blend until smooth and creamy.

3. Pour into glasses and serve immediately.

Conclusion:

These daily smoothie recipes provide a delicious and nutritious way to support your body's detoxification processes while replenishing essential nutrients and keeping you feeling energized throughout Days 2-6 of your detox journey. Experiment with different combinations of fruits, vegetables, herbs, and superfoods to create your favorite smoothie variations and enjoy the benefits of vibrant health and vitality.

CHAPTER EIGHT

Day 7: Revitalizing Smoothies to Wrap Up the Detox

As you approach the final day of your smoothie detox journey, it's time to focus on revitalizing smoothie recipes that will leave you feeling refreshed, rejuvenated, and ready to embrace life with renewed energy and vitality. These smoothies are designed to provide a final boost of nourishment and support your body's transition back to regular eating patterns. Below are three revitalizing smoothie recipes to help you wrap up your detox on a high note:

1. Green Goddess Detox Smoothie:

Ingredients:

- 1 cup spinach leaves

- 1/2 cucumber, chopped

- 1/2 green apple, cored and chopped

- 1/4 avocado, peeled and pitted

- 1 tablespoon fresh lemon juice

- 1 tablespoon fresh parsley leaves

- 1 tablespoon chia seeds

- 1 cup coconut water or almond milk

- Ice cubes (optional)

Instructions:

1. Combine all ingredients in a blender.

2. Blend until smooth and creamy.

3. Pour into glasses and serve immediately.

2. Berry Citrus Revitalizer:

Ingredients:

- 1/2 cup mixed berries (such as strawberries, blueberries, raspberries)

- 1/2 orange, peeled and segmented

- 1/2 lime, juiced

- 1 tablespoon fresh mint leaves

- 1 tablespoon chia seeds

- 1 cup coconut water or water

- Ice cubes (optional)

Instructions:

1. Place all ingredients in a blender.

2. Blend until smooth and creamy.

3. Pour into glasses and enjoy immediately.

3. Tropical Sunshine Smoothie:

Ingredients:

- 1/2 cup pineapple chunks
- 1/2 cup mango chunks
- 1/2 banana, peeled
- 1/4 cup coconut flakes
- 1 tablespoon fresh lime juice
- 1 tablespoon fresh ginger, grated
- 1 cup coconut water or almond milk
- Ice cubes (optional)

Instructions:

1. Add all ingredients to a blender.

2. Blend until smooth and creamy.

3. Pour into glasses and serve immediately.

Conclusion:

These revitalizing smoothie recipes are the perfect way to wrap up your smoothie detox journey, providing a final burst of nourishment and energy to support your body as you transition back to your regular eating patterns. Experiment with different combinations of fruits, vegetables, herbs, and superfoods to create your favorite revitalizing smoothies and celebrate the completion of your detox with a renewed sense of health and vitality.

CHAPTER NINE

Integrating Smoothie Detox into Your Lifestyle: Tips for Success

Successfully integrating smoothie detox into your lifestyle requires careful planning, commitment, and a willingness to embrace healthy habits for long-term well-being. Whether you're embarking on a short-term cleanse or incorporating smoothies into your daily routine, these tips will help you make the most of your detox experience and maintain a balanced, health-conscious lifestyle:

1. Set Clear Goals:

- Define your reasons for undertaking a smoothie detox and establish clear goals for what you hope to achieve, whether it's improved energy, weight loss, or enhanced overall health.

- Break down your goals into specific, measurable targets to track your progress and stay motivated throughout the detox process.

2. Plan Ahead:

- Take time to plan your smoothie recipes, grocery lists, and meal schedules in advance to ensure you have everything you need for a successful detox.

- Invest in quality ingredients and equipment, such as fresh fruits and vegetables, organic produce, and a high-powered blender, to maximize the nutritional benefits of your smoothies.

3. Stay Hydrated:

- In addition to consuming smoothies, prioritize hydration by drinking plenty of water throughout the day to support detoxification processes and maintain optimal hydration levels.

- Consider incorporating herbal teas, infused water, and coconut water into your hydration routine for added flavor and variety.

4. Listen to Your Body:

- Pay attention to how your body responds to the smoothie detox and adjust your approach accordingly. If you experience any adverse reactions or discomfort, consult with a healthcare professional and modify your detox plan as needed.

- Honor your hunger and fullness cues by eating regular meals and snacks in addition to consuming smoothies to ensure you're meeting your nutritional needs.

5. Practice Mindful Eating:

- Approach each smoothie with mindfulness and intention, savoring the flavors and textures while focusing on nourishing your body with wholesome ingredients.

- Take time to chew your smoothies thoroughly and pay attention to how they make you feel physically, mentally, and emotionally.

6. Incorporate Whole Foods:

- While smoothies can be a convenient way to boost nutrient intake, it's essential to complement them with whole, minimally processed foods to ensure a balanced diet.

- Include a variety of fruits, vegetables, whole grains, lean proteins, and healthy fats in your meals and snacks to provide essential nutrients and support overall health.

7. Practice Self-Care:

- Prioritize self-care practices such as adequate sleep, stress management, regular physical activity, and relaxation techniques to support your body's natural detoxification processes and promote overall well-being.

- Take time for activities that bring you joy and fulfillment, whether it's spending time outdoors, practicing yoga, or engaging in creative pursuits.

8. Gradual Transition:

- After completing a smoothie detox, gradually reintroduce solid foods into your diet to prevent digestive discomfort and support long-term dietary habits.

- Focus on incorporating nutrient-dense whole foods, such as fruits, vegetables, whole grains, and lean proteins, while minimizing processed foods, sugars, and unhealthy fats.

9. Seek Support and Accountability:

- Enlist the support of friends, family members, or a health coach to help you stay accountable to your goals and provide encouragement and motivation throughout your detox journey.

- Join online communities, support groups, or social media networks dedicated to healthy living and detoxification to connect with like-minded individuals and share experiences and tips.

10. Reflect and Reevaluate:

- Take time to reflect on your smoothie detox experience, noting any changes in your energy levels, mood, digestion, or overall well-being.

- Use this feedback to reevaluate your goals, refine your approach, and make adjustments to your lifestyle habits to continue supporting your health and vitality long after the detox is complete.

By incorporating these tips into your lifestyle, you can seamlessly integrate smoothie detox into your daily routine and reap the benefits of improved energy, vitality, and overall well-being. Remember that smoothie detox is just one component of a healthy lifestyle and should be complemented by other wellness practices to support your long-term health goals.

CHAPTER TEN

Beyond the 7 Days: Maintaining Detox Results and Incorporating Healthy Habits

Completing a smoothie detox is an accomplishment, but maintaining the results and incorporating healthy habits into your daily life are essential for long-term well-being. Transitioning from a short-term detox to a sustainable, health-conscious lifestyle requires commitment, consistency, and a holistic approach to wellness. Here are some strategies for maintaining detox results and integrating healthy habits into your life beyond the initial seven days:

1. Embrace Whole Foods:

- Continue to prioritize whole, nutrient-dense foods in your diet, including fruits, vegetables, whole grains, lean proteins, and healthy fats. These foods provide essential nutrients and support overall health and vitality.

2. Practice Balanced Eating:

- Aim for balanced meals that include a variety of macronutrients (carbohydrates, proteins, and fats) to keep you feeling satisfied and energized throughout the day. Focus on portion control and mindful eating to avoid overeating and promote digestion.

3. Hydrate Regularly:

- Maintain proper hydration by drinking plenty of water throughout the day. Aim to consume at least eight glasses of water daily, and consider incorporating hydrating beverages such as herbal teas, infused water, and coconut water into your routine.

4. Prioritize Physical Activity:

- Incorporate regular exercise into your daily routine to support overall health and well-being. Choose activities you enjoy, whether it's walking, jogging, yoga, swimming, or strength training, and aim for at least 30 minutes of moderate-intensity exercise most days of the week.

5. Manage Stress:

- Implement stress-reduction techniques such as mindfulness meditation, deep breathing exercises, yoga, or journaling to manage stress levels and promote relaxation. Prioritize self-care activities that help you unwind and recharge, such as spending time in nature, practicing hobbies, or connecting with loved ones.

6. Get Quality Sleep:

- Prioritize adequate sleep by establishing a consistent sleep schedule and creating a relaxing bedtime routine. Aim for seven to nine hours of quality sleep per night to support optimal physical and mental health.

7. Limit Toxins and Harmful Substances:

- Minimize exposure to environmental toxins, pollutants, and harmful substances such as tobacco, alcohol, and processed foods. Choose organic produce when possible, opt for natural cleaning and personal care products, and avoid smoking and excessive alcohol consumption.

8. Practice Mindful Eating:

- Cultivate mindful eating habits by paying attention to hunger and fullness cues, eating slowly, and savoring the flavors and textures of your food. Avoid distractions such as screens or multitasking during meals to promote a deeper connection with your food and enhance digestion.

9. Seek Support and Accountability:

- Surround yourself with a supportive network of friends, family members, or health professionals who share your commitment to health and wellness. Lean on them for encouragement, accountability, and motivation as you navigate your journey toward lasting health.

10. Reflect and Adjust:

- Regularly reflect on your progress, celebrate your achievements, and identify areas for improvement. Adjust your habits and routines as needed to align with your health goals and maintain momentum on your wellness journey.

By incorporating these strategies into your daily life, you can maintain the results of your smoothie detox and cultivate a sustainable, health-conscious lifestyle that supports your long-term well-being. Remember that health is a journey, not a destination, and small, consistent changes over time can lead to significant improvements in your overall health and vitality.

CHAPTER 11

DR. BARBARA'S SMOOTHIES FOR FULL-BODY DETOX

1. **Green Goddess Detox**

   - **Definition:** A rejuvenating blend of green vegetables and herbs to detoxify the body and boost energy levels.

   - **Ingredients:** Spinach, kale, cucumber, celery, parsley, lemon, ginger.

   - **Preparation:** Blend all ingredients until smooth.

   - **How to Use:** Consume in the morning on an empty stomach or as a mid-day snack.

   - **Dosage:** One serving per day.

   - **Side Effects:** Possible increase in bowel movements due to the high fiber content.

   - **Precautions:** Individuals with kidney problems should consult a healthcare professional before consuming large amounts of leafy greens.

2. **Berry Blast Detox**

- **Definition:** A fruity concoction packed with antioxidants to eliminate toxins and promote skin health.

- **Ingredients:** Mixed berries (blueberries, strawberries, raspberries), spinach, chia seeds, coconut water.

- **Preparation:** Blend berries, spinach, and coconut water until smooth, then add chia seeds and blend again briefly.

- **How to Use:** Enjoy as a refreshing breakfast or post-workout snack.

- **Dosage:** One to two servings per day.

- **Side Effects:** May cause a slight decrease in blood sugar levels.

- **Precautions:** Diabetic individuals should monitor their blood sugar levels when consuming berry-based smoothies.

3. Tropical Cleanse

- **Definition:** A tropical blend rich in enzymes and vitamins to support digestion and liver function.

- **Ingredients:** Pineapple, mango, coconut water, ginger, mint leaves.

- **Preparation:** Blend all ingredients until smooth.

- **How to Use:** Best consumed in the morning to kickstart metabolism.

- **Dosage:** One serving per day.

- **Side Effects:** Potential for gastrointestinal discomfort in individuals sensitive to acidic fruits.

- **Precautions:** Moderation is key for individuals prone to acid reflux or GERD.

4. Citrus Detox Zinger

- **Definition:** A zesty blend of citrus fruits and herbs to alkalize the body and promote hydration.

- **Ingredients:** Oranges, grapefruits, lemon, cucumber, mint leaves.

- **Preparation:** Blend all ingredients until smooth.

- **How to Use:** Ideal as a mid-day refresher or pre-workout boost.

- **Dosage:** One to two servings per day.

- **Side Effects:** Potential for tooth enamel erosion due to citrus acidity.

- **Precautions:** Rinse mouth with water after consumption to protect teeth.

5. Beetroot Cleanse

- **Definition:** A vibrant blend featuring beets to support liver detoxification and improve blood circulation.

- **Ingredients:** Beets, carrots, apple, lemon, ginger.

- **Preparation:** Blend all ingredients until smooth.

- **How to Use:** Consume post-workout for muscle recovery or as a snack.

- **Dosage:** One serving per day.

- **Side Effects:** May cause red or pink urine due to beet pigments.

- **Precautions:** Individuals prone to kidney stones should limit beet consumption.

6. Alkaline Avocado Elixir

- **Definition:** A creamy blend rich in healthy fats and alkalizing greens to balance pH levels and support detoxification.

- **Ingredients:** Avocado, spinach, cucumber, lemon, cilantro.

- **Preparation:** Blend all ingredients until smooth.

- **How to Use:** Enjoy as a nutrient-dense breakfast or post-workout recovery drink.

- **Dosage:** One serving per day.

- **Side Effects:** Unlikely, but excessive avocado consumption may lead to weight gain.

- **Precautions:** Monitor portion sizes if watching calorie intake.

7. Ginger Turmeric Tonic

- **Definition:** A warming blend infused with anti-inflammatory spices to aid digestion and support immune function.

- **Ingredients:** Turmeric root, ginger, pineapple, carrot, coconut water.

- **Preparation:** Blend all ingredients until smooth.

- **How to Use:** Consume in the morning for a natural energy boost.

- **Dosage:** One serving per day.

- **Side Effects:** Possible interactions with blood-thinning medications due to ginger and turmeric.

- **Precautions:** Consult a healthcare professional if on medication.

8. Cleansing Cucumber Mint

- **Definition:** A refreshing blend designed to hydrate and flush out toxins with cooling cucumber and mint.

- **Ingredients:** Cucumber, mint leaves, lime, coconut water.

- **Preparation:** Blend all ingredients until smooth.

- **How to Use:** Enjoy as a post-workout hydrator or mid-day pick-me-up.

- **Dosage:** One to two servings per day.

- **Side Effects:** Rare, but excessive cucumber intake may lead to bloating or gas.

- **Precautions:** Individuals with cucumber allergies should avoid this smoothie.

9. Detoxifying Dandelion Greens

- **Definition:** A bitter-sweet blend featuring dandelion greens to support liver function and aid digestion.

- **Ingredients:** Dandelion greens, cucumber, pear, lemon, parsley.

- **Preparation:** Blend all ingredients until smooth.

- **How to Use:** Consume in the morning to kickstart detoxification processes.

- **Dosage:** One serving per day.

- **Side Effects:** May cause mild gastrointestinal discomfort in sensitive individuals.

- **Precautions:** Avoid if allergic to dandelions or other members of the Asteraceae family.

10. Detoxifying Matcha Magic

- **Definition:** A vibrant blend featuring matcha green tea to boost metabolism and provide antioxidant support.

- **Ingredients:** Matcha powder, spinach, banana, almond milk, honey.

- **Preparation:** Blend all ingredients until smooth.

- **How to Use:** Enjoy as a pre-workout energizer or afternoon snack.

- **Dosage:** One serving per day.

- **Side Effects:** Excessive caffeine intake may lead to jitteriness or insomnia.

- **Precautions:** Limit consumption if sensitive to caffeine.

11. Purifying Pineapple Papaya

- **Definition:** A tropical blend rich in digestive enzymes to support gut health and aid nutrient absorption.

- **Ingredients:** Pineapple, papaya, coconut water, lime, mint leaves.

- **Preparation:** Blend all ingredients until smooth.

- **How to Use:** Consume post-meal to aid digestion or as a refreshing beverage.

- **Dosage:** One serving per day.

- **Side Effects:** Rare, but excessive bromelain intake from pineapple may cause mouth or tongue irritation.

- **Precautions:** Individuals with latex allergies may also be allergic to papaya.

12.   Chlorella Cleanse

- **Definition:** A detox powerhouse featuring chlorella algae to bind and eliminate heavy metals from the body.

- **Ingredients:** Chlorella powder, cucumber, apple, lemon, ginger.

- **Preparation:** Blend all ingredients until smooth.

- **How to Use:** Best consumed in the morning on an empty stomach for maximum absorption.

- **Dosage:** One serving per day.

- **Side Effects:** Potential for gastrointestinal discomfort due to chlorella's detoxifying effects.

- **Precautions:** Start with small doses to assess tolerance, and avoid if allergic to seafood.

13.   Spicy Cayenne Cleanse

- **Definition:** A fiery blend featuring cayenne pepper to boost metabolism and stimulate circulation.

- **Ingredients:** Cayenne pepper, lemon, apple, cucumber, spinach.

- **Preparation:** Blend all ingredients until smooth.

- **How to Use:** Consume in the morning for a metabolism kickstart or as a pre-workout energizer.

- **Dosage:** One serving per day.

- **Side Effects:** May cause temporary discomfort due to cayenne's heat.

- **Precautions:** Avoid if sensitive to spicy foods or if prone to digestive issues like acid reflux.

14. **Charcoal Cleanse**

- **Definition:** A detoxifying blend featuring activated charcoal to absorb toxins and promote gut health.

- **Ingredients:** Activated charcoal powder, coconut water, pineapple, banana, spinach.

- **Preparation:** Blend all ingredients until smooth.

- **How to Use:** Consume as needed to alleviate bloating or digestive discomfort.

- **Dosage:** One serving per day or as directed by a healthcare professional.

- **Side Effects:** May cause darkened stools due to charcoal's coloring properties.

- **Precautions:** Take charcoal supplements away from medications, as it may interfere with absorption.

15.   Blue Majik Detox

- **Definition:** A vibrant blue blend featuring spirulina to provide antioxidant support and promote detoxification.

- **Ingredients:** Blue spirulina powder, banana, pineapple, coconut water, spinach.

- **Preparation:** Blend all ingredients until smooth.

- **How to Use:** Enjoy as a post-workout recovery drink or as a refreshing beverage.

- **Dosage:** One serving per day.

- **Side Effects:** Rare, but spirulina may cause allergic reactions in sensitive individuals.

- **Precautions:** Start with small doses to assess tolerance, and avoid if allergic to seafood.

Charcoal Detox:

Definition: Charcoal detox refers to the use of activated charcoal, typically derived from sources like coconut shells or bamboo, to help remove toxins and impurities from the body. Activated charcoal is known for its highly porous surface, which allows it to trap toxins and chemicals.

Ingredients: Activated charcoal is the primary ingredient used in charcoal detox. It's available in various forms, including powder, capsules, and tablets.

How to Prepare: Preparing for a charcoal detox involves selecting the appropriate form of activated charcoal and following the recommended dosage instructions provided on the product packaging or as directed by a healthcare provider.

Dosage: The dosage of activated charcoal for detoxification purposes varies depending on factors such as the individual's weight, age, and overall health status. It's essential to follow the recommended dosage instructions carefully to avoid potential side effects.

How to Use: Activated charcoal can be consumed orally by mixing it with water or other liquids, or it may be taken in capsule or tablet form. It's typically taken on an empty stomach, either between meals or several hours before or after eating, to maximize its detoxifying effects. Activated charcoal can also be used topically in skincare products to absorb excess oil and impurities from the skin.

Side Effects: While activated charcoal is generally considered safe for short-term use, it may cause side effects such as constipation, black stools, or gastrointestinal discomfort in some individuals. It's essential to drink plenty of water when consuming activated charcoal to prevent dehydration and ensure proper elimination of toxins from the body. Activated charcoal may also interfere with the absorption of certain medications, so it's advisable to take it at least two hours before or after taking any medications. Individuals with gastrointestinal conditions, such as blockages or bleeding, should avoid using activated charcoal without consulting with a healthcare provider.

Chlorella Supplements:

Definition: Chlorella supplements are derived from a type of single-celled green algae called Chlorella vulgaris. They are known for their high nutrient content, including vitamins, minerals, antioxidants, and amino acids.

Ingredients: Chlorella supplements contain dried and processed Chlorella vulgaris algae. They may be available in various forms, including tablets, capsules, powders, and liquid extracts.

How to Prepare: Preparing for chlorella supplementation involves selecting the desired form of the supplement and following the recommended dosage instructions provided on the product packaging or as advised by a healthcare provider.

Dosage: The dosage of chlorella supplements varies depending on factors such as the individual's age, weight, and health goals. It's essential to follow the recommended dosage instructions to ensure safety and effectiveness.

How to Use: Chlorella supplements can be consumed orally by swallowing tablets or capsules with water, or they may be mixed into smoothies, juices, or other beverages. Some people also use chlorella powder to sprinkle on food or incorporate into recipes. Chlorella supplements are typically taken once or twice daily with meals.

Side Effects: Chlorella supplements are generally well-tolerated by most people when taken in recommended doses. However, some individuals may experience mild side effects such as digestive upset, including nausea, diarrhea, or flatulence. These side effects are usually temporary and subside with continued use or by adjusting the dosage. Chlorella supplements may also cause allergic reactions in some individuals, particularly those with sensitivities to algae or seafood. It's advisable to start with a low dose and monitor for any adverse reactions. Individuals with certain medical conditions or who are pregnant or breastfeeding should consult with a healthcare provider before starting chlorella supplementation.

Colon Cleansing:

Definition: Colon cleansing, also known as colonic irrigation or colon hydrotherapy, is a practice aimed at removing toxins and waste buildup from the colon. It typically involves flushing the colon with water or other substances to stimulate bowel movements and promote detoxification.

Ingredients: Colon cleansing procedures may use various ingredients, including water, herbal solutions, saline solutions, or other substances designed to soften stool and facilitate elimination.

How to Prepare: Preparing for a colon cleansing procedure may involve dietary restrictions, such as avoiding solid foods for a period before the procedure, and ensuring proper hydration. It's essential to follow any instructions provided by the healthcare provider or practitioner performing the colon cleansing.

Dosage: The frequency and duration of colon cleansing procedures vary depending on factors such as individual health goals and the specific method used. Some people may undergo colon cleansing as a one-time treatment, while others may incorporate it into a regular detoxification regimen.

How to Use: Colon cleansing procedures may be performed by healthcare professionals in clinical settings or by using at-home kits. During the procedure, a tube is inserted into the rectum, and water or a cleansing solution is gently introduced into the colon to flush out waste material. The process typically takes about 45 minutes to an hour.

Side Effects: While colon cleansing may offer temporary relief from symptoms such as constipation or bloating, it's important to note that it's not necessary for everyone and may carry risks. Potential side effects of colon cleansing include dehydration, electrolyte imbalance, perforation of the colon, infection, and disruption of the natural balance of bacteria in the gut. Colon cleansing may also interfere with the body's natural bowel function and lead to dependence on laxatives for regular bowel movements. Individuals considering colon cleansing should consult with a healthcare provider to weigh the potential benefits and risks.

Cranberry Juice:

Definition: Cranberry juice is a tart and tangy beverage made from the juice of cranberries, which are small, red berries known for their high antioxidant content and potential health benefits.

Ingredients: Cranberry juice is made primarily from cranberries, which contain vitamins, minerals, antioxidants, and phytonutrients such as flavonoids and polyphenols.

How to Prepare: Commercially available cranberry juice is typically prepared by pressing or crushing cranberries to extract the juice, which may be further processed and filtered to remove pulp and solids. Some varieties of cranberry juice may contain added sugars or other ingredients for flavor enhancement.

Dosage: There isn't a specific dosage for cranberry juice, but incorporating it into your diet in moderation can provide potential health benefits. Drinking one to two glasses of cranberry juice per day is often recommended for urinary tract health.

How to Use: Cranberry juice can be consumed on its own as a refreshing beverage or mixed with other juices or water. Some people also use cranberry juice as an ingredient in cocktails, smoothies, or salad dressings. It's essential to choose unsweetened cranberry juice or opt for varieties with minimal added sugars to maximize the health benefits.

Side Effects: While cranberry juice is generally safe for most people when consumed in moderation, some individuals may experience side effects such as gastrointestinal upset or diarrhea, particularly if consumed in large quantities. Cranberry juice may also interact with certain medications, such as blood thinners, and individuals with a history of kidney stones may need to limit their intake due to the high oxalate content of cranberries. It's advisable to consult with a healthcare provider before incorporating cranberry juice into your diet, especially if you have underlying health conditions or are taking medications.

Detox Baths:

Definition: Detox baths are a form of hydrotherapy that involves soaking in a bath containing various ingredients believed to help remove toxins from the body, promote relaxation, and support overall well-being.

Ingredients: Detox baths may include a variety of ingredients such as Epsom salts, baking soda, essential oils, apple cider vinegar, bentonite clay, ginger, and herbs like lavender or chamomile.

How to Prepare: Preparing a detox bath involves adding the desired ingredients to a bathtub filled with warm water. The water temperature should be comfortable for soaking, and the ingredients should be thoroughly mixed into the water to ensure even distribution.

Dosage: There isn't a specific dosage for detox baths, as the frequency and duration of soaking can vary depending on individual preferences and needs. Some people may enjoy a detox bath once a week as part of their self-care routine, while others may choose to soak more or less frequently.

How to Use: To use a detox bath, simply immerse yourself in the tub and soak for 20 to 30 minutes or longer, allowing the ingredients to work their magic. It's essential to relax and breathe deeply during the bath to enhance the calming effects. After soaking, rinse off with clean water and pat dry with a towel.

Side Effects: Detox baths are generally safe for most people when used as directed, but some individuals may experience skin irritation or allergic reactions to certain ingredients. It's essential to perform a patch test before using new ingredients and discontinue use if any adverse reactions occur. Additionally, pregnant or breastfeeding women, individuals with certain medical conditions, or those taking medications should consult with a healthcare provider before using detox baths.

Detox Teas:

Definition: Detox teas are herbal teas or blends formulated with ingredients believed to support the body's detoxification processes, aid digestion, promote weight loss, and boost overall health.

Ingredients: Detox teas may contain a variety of ingredients such as green tea, dandelion, milk thistle, ginger, licorice root, peppermint, cinnamon, and various herbs and botanicals known for their detoxifying and digestive properties.

How to Prepare: Preparing detox tea involves steeping the tea bag or loose tea leaves in hot water for several minutes, typically 5 to 10 minutes, to allow the flavors and beneficial compounds to infuse into the water. Some detox teas may be consumed hot or cold, depending on personal preference.

Dosage: The recommended dosage of detox tea can vary depending on the specific blend and individual tolerance. It's generally advisable to start with a single cup per day and gradually increase as desired, following the instructions provided on the tea packaging.

How to Use: Detox teas can be enjoyed at any time of day, but many people prefer to drink them in the morning or before meals to support digestion and metabolism. It's essential to listen to your body's cues and adjust the frequency of consumption based on how you feel.

Side Effects: While detox teas are generally considered safe for most people when consumed in moderation, some individuals may experience side effects such as gastrointestinal upset, including bloating, gas, or diarrhea, especially if sensitive to certain ingredients. Detox teas containing caffeine may also cause jitteriness or disrupt sleep in some individuals. It's important to read the ingredient list carefully and avoid detox teas containing ingredients that may interact with medications or exacerbate underlying health conditions. Pregnant or breastfeeding women, individuals with certain medical conditions, or those taking medications should consult with a healthcare provider before using detox teas.

Dry Skin Brushing:

Definition: Dry skin brushing is a self-care technique that involves using a natural bristle brush to gently massage the skin in a specific pattern to promote exfoliation, stimulate circulation, and support lymphatic drainage.

Ingredients: Dry skin brushing requires a natural bristle brush with a long handle for reaching all areas of the body.

How to Prepare: Preparing for dry skin brushing involves selecting a suitable brush with natural bristles and ensuring that the skin is dry and free from moisturizers or oils.

Dosage: There isn't a specific dosage for dry skin brushing, but it's generally recommended to brush the skin for a few minutes each day, preferably before bathing or showering, to reap the benefits.

How to Use: To use a dry skin brush, start at the feet and brush upwards towards the heart using gentle, circular motions. Continue brushing each area of the body, including the legs, arms, back, and abdomen, for several minutes. Avoid brushing over sensitive or broken skin areas.

Side Effects: Dry skin brushing is generally safe for most people when done correctly, but it may cause skin irritation or sensitivity in some individuals, especially those with sensitive skin or conditions such as eczema or psoriasis. It's essential to use gentle pressure and avoid brushing over areas of inflamed or broken skin. If irritation occurs, discontinue use and consult with a dermatologist.

Epsom Salt Baths:

Definition: Epsom salt baths involve adding Epsom salt, also known as magnesium sulfate, to a warm bath to help soothe sore muscles, relieve stress, promote relaxation, and potentially detoxify the body.

Ingredients: Epsom salt is the primary ingredient used in Epsom salt baths. It's a naturally occurring mineral compound composed of magnesium, sulfur, and oxygen.

How to Prepare: Preparing for an Epsom salt bath involves adding the desired amount of Epsom salt to a bathtub filled with warm water. The water temperature should be comfortable for soaking, and the Epsom salt should be thoroughly dissolved before entering the bath.

Dosage: The recommended dosage of Epsom salt for a bath can vary depending on individual preferences and needs. As a general guideline, adding 1 to 2 cups of Epsom salt to a standard-sized bathtub filled with warm water is typically sufficient for most people.

How to Use: To use an Epsom salt bath, simply immerse yourself in the tub and soak for 20 to 30 minutes or longer, allowing the Epsom salt to dissolve and infuse into the water. It's essential to relax and breathe deeply during the bath to maximize the calming effects. After soaking, rinse off with clean water and pat dry with a towel.

Side Effects: Epsom salt baths are generally safe for most people when used as directed, but some individuals may experience skin irritation or allergic reactions to Epsom salt. It's essential to perform a patch test before using Epsom salt baths and discontinue use if any adverse reactions occur. Pregnant or breastfeeding women, individuals with certain medical conditions, or those taking medications should consult with a healthcare provider before using Epsom salt baths. Additionally, it's important to stay hydrated during and after an Epsom salt bath to prevent dehydration.

Exercise:

Definition: Exercise refers to physical activity performed to improve health, fitness, or overall well-being. It encompasses a wide range of activities, including cardiovascular exercises, strength training, flexibility exercises, and balance exercises.

Ingredients: Exercise requires varying combinations of movements, depending on the specific type of activity. Examples include running, walking, cycling, swimming, weightlifting, yoga, Pilates, and dancing.

How to Prepare: Preparing for exercise involves selecting appropriate clothing and footwear, warming up with dynamic stretches or light cardio, and ensuring hydration and nutrition levels are adequate.

Dosage: The recommended dosage of exercise depends on factors such as age, fitness level, health status, and exercise goals. As a general guideline, adults should aim for at least 150 minutes of moderate-intensity aerobic activity or 75 minutes of vigorous-intensity aerobic activity per week, along with muscle-strengthening activities on two or more days per week.

How to Use: Exercise can be integrated into daily routines in various ways, such as walking or cycling for transportation, taking the stairs instead of the elevator, or participating in structured exercise sessions at a gym or fitness facility. It's important to choose activities that are enjoyable and sustainable to maintain long-term adherence.

Side Effects: While exercise offers numerous health benefits, including improved cardiovascular health, weight management, mood enhancement, and stress reduction, overexertion or improper technique can lead to injuries such as strains, sprains, or fractures. It's essential to listen to your body, start gradually, and seek guidance from qualified fitness professionals to minimize the risk of injury.

Fasting:

Definition: Fasting involves voluntarily abstaining from food and/or drink for a specified period, often for religious, spiritual, health, or weight loss purposes.

Ingredients: Fasting requires no specific ingredients, as it involves restricting food intake for a predetermined period.

How to Prepare: Preparing for a fast involves planning the duration and type of fast, ensuring adequate hydration, and considering any potential medical implications or contraindications.

Dosage: The duration and frequency of fasting can vary widely, ranging from intermittent fasting protocols lasting several hours to extended fasts lasting multiple days or weeks. It's essential to choose a fasting regimen that aligns with individual health goals and preferences and to consult with a healthcare professional if there are any concerns.

How to Use: Fasting protocols may involve various approaches, including intermittent fasting (e.g., 16/8 method, alternate-day fasting), time-restricted feeding, water fasting, juice fasting, or religious fasting practices. It's important to stay hydrated during fasting periods and to break the fast gradually to avoid digestive discomfort.

Side Effects: While fasting may offer potential health benefits such as improved metabolic health, weight loss, and cellular repair processes, it can also pose risks, especially for certain populations such as pregnant or breastfeeding women, individuals with medical conditions such as diabetes or eating disorders, and those taking medications. Side effects of fasting may include dehydration, low blood sugar, headaches, dizziness, fatigue, irritability, and difficulty concentrating. It's essential to approach fasting mindfully, listen to your body's cues, and seek guidance from a healthcare professional before embarking on any fasting regimen, particularly if you have underlying health concerns.

Foot Detox Pads:

Definition: Foot detox pads are adhesive patches that are applied to the soles of the feet overnight. They are believed to help draw out toxins from the body through the feet while you sleep, promoting detoxification and overall wellness.

Ingredients: Foot detox pads typically contain a combination of natural ingredients such as bamboo vinegar, tourmaline, herbs (e.g., ginger, lavender, mint), and other botanical extracts. These ingredients are believed to have detoxifying properties and help absorb toxins from the body.

How to Prepare: Preparing for foot detox pad application involves cleansing and drying the feet thoroughly before bedtime. The pads are then applied to the soles of the feet, preferably on the reflexology points, and left on overnight.

Dosage: The frequency of foot detox pad use can vary depending on individual preferences and needs. Some people may use them nightly, while others may use them a few times a week or less frequently.

How to Use: To use foot detox pads, simply adhere them to the clean, dry soles of your feet before bedtime. Wear socks over the pads to keep them in place overnight. In the morning, remove the pads and discard them. Some pads may change color or appear darker after use, which is often attributed to the absorption of toxins from the body.

Side Effects: While foot detox pads are generally considered safe for most people, some individuals may experience skin irritation or allergic reactions to certain ingredients in the pads. It's essential to perform a patch test before using foot detox pads extensively and discontinue use if any adverse reactions occur. Additionally, foot detox pads may not be suitable for individuals with sensitive skin or certain medical conditions, so it's advisable to consult with a healthcare provider before using them, especially if you have concerns.

Herbal Detox Supplements:

Definition: Herbal detox supplements are dietary supplements formulated with a combination of herbs and botanical extracts believed to support the body's detoxification processes, promote liver health, and eliminate toxins.

Ingredients: Herbal detox supplements may contain a variety of ingredients, including milk thistle, dandelion root, burdock root, turmeric, artichoke extract, schisandra berry, and other herbs known for their detoxifying and liver-supportive properties. These supplements may be available in various forms, including capsules, tablets, powders, or liquid extracts.

How to Prepare: Preparing for herbal detox supplement use involves selecting a reputable product from a trusted manufacturer and following the recommended dosage instructions provided on the product packaging or as advised by a healthcare provider.

Dosage: The recommended dosage of herbal detox supplements can vary depending on the specific formulation and individual needs. It's essential to follow the dosage instructions carefully and not exceed the recommended dose without consulting with a healthcare provider.

How to Use: Herbal detox supplements are typically taken orally with water or another beverage, preferably with meals to enhance absorption and minimize gastrointestinal upset. Some supplements may recommend a specific dosing schedule or additional dietary and lifestyle recommendations to support detoxification.

Side Effects: While herbal detox supplements are generally well-tolerated by most people when used as directed, some individuals may experience side effects such as gastrointestinal upset, allergic reactions, or interactions with medications. It's essential to read the ingredient list carefully and avoid supplements containing ingredients that may trigger allergic reactions or interact with medications you're taking. Pregnant or breastfeeding women, individuals with certain medical conditions, or those taking medications should consult with a healthcare provider before using herbal detox supplements. Additionally, it's important to remember that dietary supplements are not regulated as strictly as pharmaceutical drugs, so quality and safety can vary between products. Choose supplements from reputable brands with third-party testing and certifications to ensure product quality and purity.

Hydrotherapy:

Definition: Hydrotherapy is a therapeutic approach that involves using water at varying temperatures and pressures to promote health and well-being. It encompasses a wide range of techniques, including hot baths, cold plunges, steam baths, saunas, whirlpools, and water exercises.

Ingredients: Hydrotherapy typically requires water and may involve additional ingredients such as essential oils, Epsom salt, herbal infusions, or other substances added to enhance the therapeutic effects.

How to Prepare: Preparing for hydrotherapy involves selecting the appropriate technique based on individual needs and preferences, ensuring that the water temperature and conditions are safe and comfortable, and following any specific instructions provided for the chosen method.

Dosage: The frequency and duration of hydrotherapy sessions can vary depending on the specific technique used, individual health goals, and response to treatment. Some people may benefit from regular hydrotherapy sessions as part of a holistic health regimen, while others may use hydrotherapy occasionally for relaxation or symptom relief.

How to Use: Hydrotherapy techniques can be incorporated into daily routines or used as standalone treatments. For example, a warm bath with Epsom salt may be used to soothe sore muscles, while a cold plunge or contrast shower may be used to invigorate and energize the body. It's essential to listen to your body's cues and adjust the intensity and duration of hydrotherapy sessions as needed.

Side Effects: Hydrotherapy is generally safe for most people when used appropriately, but it may not be suitable for everyone, especially those with certain medical conditions or sensitivities to temperature extremes. Potential side effects of hydrotherapy may include dehydration, dizziness, fainting, skin irritation, or exacerbation of existing health issues. It's important to consult with a healthcare provider before starting hydrotherapy, especially if you have underlying health concerns or are taking medications.

Juice Fasting:

Definition: Juice fasting, also known as juice cleansing or juice detoxification, involves consuming only fruit and vegetable juices for a specified period while abstaining from solid foods. It's often done as a short-term dietary cleanse or detox to eliminate toxins, promote weight loss, and improve overall health.

Ingredients: Juice fasting requires fresh fruits and vegetables, preferably organic, and a juicer or blender to extract the juice. Common ingredients used in juice fasting include leafy greens, carrots, celery, cucumbers, apples, beets, ginger, and citrus fruits.

How to Prepare: Preparing for a juice fast involves selecting a variety of fruits and vegetables, washing them thoroughly, and juicing them to extract the liquid. It's important to drink freshly prepared juices immediately to retain their nutritional value and minimize exposure to air and light, which can degrade certain nutrients.

Dosage: The duration of a juice fast can vary depending on individual goals and preferences. Some people may choose to fast for a few days, while others may extend the fast for a week or longer. It's essential to listen to your body's cues and break the fast if you experience significant discomfort or adverse effects.

How to Use: During a juice fast, participants typically consume freshly prepared fruit and vegetable juices throughout the day, drinking them at regular intervals to maintain hydration and energy levels. It's important to drink plenty of water in addition to juice to prevent dehydration and support detoxification processes.

Side Effects: While juice fasting may offer potential health benefits such as weight loss, improved digestion, and increased energy levels, it can also pose risks, especially if done for an extended period or without proper guidance. Potential side effects of juice fasting may include nutrient deficiencies, blood sugar fluctuations, dizziness, fatigue, headaches, and gastrointestinal upset. Juice fasting may not be suitable for everyone, especially those with certain medical conditions such as diabetes, kidney disease, or eating disorders. It's important to consult with a healthcare provider or registered dietitian before starting a juice fast, especially if you have underlying health concerns or are taking medications. Additionally, it's advisable to transition gradually into and out of a juice fast to minimize digestive discomfort and support long-term dietary changes.

Lemon Water:

Definition: Lemon water is a beverage made by squeezing fresh lemon juice into water. It's commonly consumed for its refreshing taste and potential health benefits.

Ingredients: Lemon water requires fresh lemon juice and water. Some people may also add additional ingredients such as honey, mint, or ginger for flavor enhancement.

How to Prepare: Preparing lemon water involves squeezing the juice of one or more fresh lemons into a glass of water and stirring to combine. The ratio of lemon juice to water can be adjusted according to personal taste preferences.

Dosage: There isn't a specific dosage for lemon water, but incorporating it into your daily routine can provide potential health benefits. Aim to drink one or more glasses of lemon water per day, preferably on an empty stomach in the morning or throughout the day for hydration and refreshment.

How to Use: Lemon water can be enjoyed cold, at room temperature, or warm, depending on personal preference. It can be consumed as a standalone beverage or incorporated into other drinks such as teas or smoothies. Some people also use lemon water as a flavor enhancer for cooking or salad dressings.

Side Effects: Lemon water is generally well-tolerated by most people when consumed in moderation. However, some individuals may experience side effects such as heartburn, acid reflux, or tooth erosion due to the acidic nature of lemon juice. It's important to rinse your mouth with plain water after drinking lemon water and avoid brushing your teeth immediately to protect tooth enamel. If you have specific health concerns or dietary restrictions, consult with a healthcare provider or registered dietitian before making significant changes to your diet.

Lymphatic Drainage Massage:

Definition: Lymphatic drainage massage is a specialized massage technique designed to stimulate the lymphatic system and encourage the natural flow of lymph fluid throughout the body. It's often used to reduce swelling, promote detoxification, boost immunity, and support overall health and well-being.

Ingredients: Lymphatic drainage massage requires no specific ingredients, as it involves manual manipulation of the skin and underlying tissues to stimulate lymphatic circulation. However, some therapists may use a gentle massage oil or lotion to reduce friction and enhance the massage experience.

How to Prepare: Preparing for a lymphatic drainage massage involves selecting a qualified massage therapist trained in lymphatic drainage techniques and scheduling a session. It's important to communicate any health concerns or preferences with the therapist before the massage begins.

Dosage: The frequency and duration of lymphatic drainage massage sessions can vary depending on individual needs and goals. Some people may benefit from regular sessions to address specific health issues, while others may use lymphatic drainage massage occasionally for relaxation or maintenance.

How to Use: During a lymphatic drainage massage, the therapist uses gentle, rhythmic movements to stimulate lymphatic circulation and encourage the removal of toxins and waste products from the body. The massage may focus on specific areas of the body, such as the arms, legs, abdomen, or face, depending on individual needs and concerns.

Side Effects: Lymphatic drainage massage is generally safe for most people when performed by a qualified therapist. However, some individuals may experience mild side effects such as temporary soreness, fatigue, or increased urination following a massage session. These side effects are usually temporary and subside with time. If you have specific health conditions such as cancer, lymphedema, or circulatory disorders, or if you're pregnant, it's essential to consult with a healthcare provider before undergoing lymphatic drainage massage to ensure it's safe and appropriate for you.

Milk Thistle Supplements:

Definition: Milk thistle supplements are dietary supplements made from the seeds of the milk thistle plant (Silybum marianum). They are known for their potential liver-supportive properties and are commonly used to promote liver health and detoxification.

Ingredients: Milk thistle supplements typically contain extracts from the seeds of the milk thistle plant, standardized to contain a specific amount of the active compound silymarin. Other ingredients may include fillers, binders, and additional herbs or botanicals.

How to Prepare: Preparing for milk thistle supplement use involves selecting a reputable product from a trusted manufacturer and following the recommended dosage instructions provided on the product packaging or as advised by a healthcare provider.

Dosage: The recommended dosage of milk thistle supplements can vary depending on the specific formulation and individual needs. It's essential to follow the dosage instructions carefully and not exceed the recommended dose without consulting with a healthcare provider.

How to Use: Milk thistle supplements are typically taken orally with water or another beverage, preferably with meals to enhance absorption and minimize gastrointestinal upset. Some supplements may recommend a specific dosing schedule or additional dietary and lifestyle recommendations to support liver health and detoxification.

Side Effects: Milk thistle supplements are generally well-tolerated by most people when used as directed, but some individuals may experience side effects such as gastrointestinal upset, allergic reactions, or interactions with medications. It's essential to read the ingredient list carefully and avoid supplements containing ingredients that may trigger allergic reactions or interact with medications you're taking. Pregnant or breastfeeding women, individuals with certain medical conditions, or those taking medications should consult with a healthcare provider before using milk thistle supplements. Additionally, it's important to choose supplements from reputable brands with third-party testing and certifications to ensure product quality and purity.

Oil Pulling:

Definition: Oil pulling is an ancient Ayurvedic practice that involves swishing oil around in the mouth for a specified period, typically 10 to 20 minutes, to promote oral health and detoxification.

Ingredients: Oil pulling requires a natural oil such as coconut oil, sesame oil, or sunflower oil. These oils are believed to have antimicrobial properties and may help remove bacteria, plaque, and toxins from the mouth.

How to Prepare: Preparing for oil pulling involves selecting a suitable oil and ensuring that it's in liquid form, preferably at room temperature. Some people may choose to add a few drops of essential oil, such as peppermint or tea tree oil, for flavor or additional benefits.

Dosage: The recommended duration for oil pulling is typically 10 to 20 minutes, although some people may choose to swish the oil for longer periods. It's important to start with a shorter duration, such as 5 minutes, and gradually increase the time as you become accustomed to the practice.

How to Use: To perform oil pulling, take a tablespoon of oil and swish it around in your mouth, making sure to pull it through your teeth and around your gums. Avoid swallowing the oil, as it may contain bacteria and toxins removed from the mouth. After the designated time, spit out the oil into a trash bin and rinse your mouth thoroughly with water.

Side Effects: Oil pulling is generally safe for most people when done correctly, but some individuals may experience side effects such as nausea, upset stomach, or a gag reflex when swishing the oil. These side effects are typically mild and temporary and may subside with continued practice. If you experience any discomfort or adverse reactions, discontinue oil pulling and consult with a healthcare provider. Additionally, oil pulling is not a substitute for regular oral hygiene practices such as brushing and flossing, so it's important to continue these habits for optimal oral health.

Oxygen Therapy:

Definition: Oxygen therapy is a medical treatment that involves administering supplemental oxygen to individuals with breathing difficulties or low blood oxygen levels. It's used to improve oxygen delivery to tissues and organs, relieve symptoms of hypoxemia (low blood oxygen), and support respiratory function.

Ingredients: Oxygen therapy typically requires medical-grade oxygen, which is administered using various delivery systems such as nasal cannulas, oxygen masks, or oxygen concentrators. The oxygen itself is the active ingredient in this therapy.

How to Prepare: Preparing for oxygen therapy involves assessing the individual's oxygen needs, determining the appropriate flow rate and delivery system, and ensuring access to medical-grade oxygen and necessary equipment.

Dosage: The dosage of oxygen therapy is prescribed by a healthcare provider based on factors such as the severity of hypoxemia, underlying health conditions, and individual oxygen requirements. Oxygen flow rates are measured in liters per minute (LPM), and the prescribed flow rate may vary depending on the specific situation.

How to Use: Oxygen therapy is typically administered under the guidance of healthcare professionals, either in a hospital setting, outpatient clinic, or at home. The delivery system and flow rate are adjusted as needed to maintain adequate blood oxygen levels and relieve symptoms of hypoxemia.

Side Effects: While oxygen therapy is generally safe and well-tolerated when used as prescribed, excessive oxygen supplementation can lead to complications such as oxygen toxicity, respiratory depression, and absorption atelectasis (collapse of lung tissue). It's essential to follow the prescribed oxygen flow rate and usage instructions carefully and to monitor for signs of oxygen toxicity or respiratory distress. Individuals with certain respiratory conditions such as chronic obstructive pulmonary disease (COPD) may require careful monitoring and adjustment of oxygen therapy to prevent complications.

Probiotic Supplements:

Definition: Probiotic supplements are dietary supplements containing live bacteria or yeasts that are believed to provide health benefits by restoring or maintaining a healthy balance of gut microbiota (the community of microorganisms in the digestive tract).

Ingredients: Probiotic supplements contain various strains of beneficial bacteria or yeasts, such as Lactobacillus, Bifidobacterium, Saccharomyces, or Streptococcus. These microorganisms are typically present in fermented foods like yogurt, kefir, sauerkraut, and kimchi.

How to Prepare: Preparing for probiotic supplement use involves selecting a suitable product from a reputable manufacturer and following the recommended dosage instructions provided on the product packaging or as advised by a healthcare provider.

Dosage: The recommended dosage of probiotic supplements can vary depending on the specific formulation, strain, and individual needs. It's essential to follow the dosage instructions carefully and to choose a supplement with strains and doses supported by scientific evidence for the intended health benefits.

How to Use: Probiotic supplements are typically taken orally with water or another beverage, preferably with meals to enhance absorption and minimize gastrointestinal upset. Some supplements may recommend refrigeration to maintain the viability of live probiotic cultures.

Side Effects: Probiotic supplements are generally safe for most people when used as directed, but some individuals may experience side effects such as bloating, gas, diarrhea, or abdominal discomfort, especially when first starting probiotic supplementation or with high doses. These side effects are usually mild and temporary and may subside with continued use. It's important to choose probiotic supplements from reputable brands with third-party testing and certifications to ensure product quality and potency. Individuals with certain medical conditions, compromised immune systems, or allergies to specific probiotic strains should consult with a healthcare provider before using probiotic supplements. Additionally, probiotic supplements are not a substitute for a balanced diet and healthy lifestyle, so it's essential to focus on overall dietary patterns and gut health practices for optimal well-being.

Raw Food Diet:

Definition: A raw food diet is a dietary approach that emphasizes consuming uncooked, unprocessed, and predominantly plant-based foods. It's based on the belief that cooking destroys enzymes, vitamins, and other nutrients in food and that consuming raw foods can promote better health and vitality.

Ingredients: A raw food diet includes a variety of fruits, vegetables, nuts, seeds, sprouted grains, legumes, and seaweed. Common raw food staples include salads, smoothies, raw fruits and vegetables, nuts and seeds, raw dairy products (such as unpasteurized milk and cheese), and fermented foods (such as sauerkraut and kimchi).

How to Prepare: Preparing for a raw food diet involves selecting fresh, organic, and preferably locally sourced ingredients. Food is typically eaten raw or minimally processed, such as juicing, blending, soaking, sprouting, or dehydrating at low temperatures to preserve nutrients.

Dosage: There isn't a specific dosage for a raw food diet, as it depends on individual preferences, nutritional needs, and health goals. Some people may choose to follow a fully raw diet, while others may incorporate raw foods into their diet alongside cooked foods.

How to Use: On a raw food diet, food is consumed in its natural state, with minimal processing or cooking. This may include eating raw fruits and vegetables, salads, smoothies, raw nuts and seeds, and raw dairy products. It's important to practice food safety and hygiene when handling raw foods to prevent contamination and foodborne illness.

Side Effects: While a raw food diet can provide numerous health benefits such as increased consumption of vitamins, minerals, fiber, and antioxidants, it can also pose risks if not balanced properly. Potential side effects of a raw food diet may include nutrient deficiencies (such as vitamin B12, iron, calcium, and protein), digestive issues (such as bloating, gas, and diarrhea), and foodborne illness from consuming raw or undercooked foods. It's essential to plan meals carefully to ensure adequate nutrient intake and to listen to your body's cues to prevent deficiencies or imbalances. Individuals with certain health conditions, such as gastrointestinal disorders or compromised immune systems, should consult with a healthcare provider or registered dietitian before starting a raw food diet.

Skin Detox Masks:

Definition: Skin detox masks, also known as detoxifying facial masks or purifying face masks, are skincare products designed to remove impurities, excess oil, and toxins from the skin, leaving it feeling clean, refreshed, and revitalized.

Ingredients: Skin detox masks may contain a variety of ingredients chosen for their detoxifying, purifying, and clarifying properties. Common ingredients include clay (such as kaolin or bentonite), charcoal, activated charcoal, mud, seaweed, herbal extracts, antioxidants, and essential oils.

How to Prepare: Preparing for a skin detox mask involves selecting a suitable product based on skin type and concerns. Some masks come in pre-packaged single-use packets or jars, while others may be mixed with water or another liquid to form a paste before application.

Dosage: The frequency of skin detox mask application can vary depending on individual skin needs and preferences. Some people may use a detox mask once or twice a week as part of their skincare routine, while others may use them less frequently or as needed.

How to Use: To use a skin detox mask, apply a thin, even layer to clean, dry skin, avoiding the eye area and lips. Allow the mask to dry completely, typically for 10 to 20 minutes, before rinsing it off with warm water. Follow up with a moisturizer or other skincare products as needed.

Side Effects: Skin detox masks are generally safe for most people when used as directed, but some individuals may experience skin irritation, redness, or dryness, especially if they have sensitive skin or allergies to certain ingredients. It's essential to perform a patch test before using a new detox mask and to discontinue use if any adverse reactions occur. Additionally, overuse of detox masks or leaving them on for too long can lead to excessive dryness or irritation, so it's important to follow package instructions and listen to your skin's needs. If you have specific skin concerns or medical conditions, consult with a dermatologist or skincare professional before incorporating detox masks into your skincare routine.

Spirulina Supplements:

Definition: Spirulina supplements are dietary supplements made from spirulina, a type of blue-green algae that grows in freshwater lakes, rivers, and ponds. Spirulina is known for its dense nutritional profile and is often consumed as a source of protein, vitamins, minerals, antioxidants, and other beneficial compounds.

Ingredients: Spirulina supplements contain dried spirulina algae, typically in powdered or tablet form. Spirulina is rich in nutrients such as protein, vitamins (including B vitamins and vitamin K), minerals (such as iron, calcium, magnesium, and potassium), antioxidants (including phycocyanin and beta-carotene), and essential fatty acids.

How to Prepare: Preparing for spirulina supplement use involves selecting a reputable product from a trusted manufacturer and following the recommended dosage instructions provided on the product packaging or as advised by a healthcare provider.

Dosage: The recommended dosage of spirulina supplements can vary depending on the specific formulation and individual needs. It's essential to follow the dosage instructions carefully and not exceed the recommended dose without consulting with a healthcare provider.

How to Use: Spirulina supplements are typically taken orally with water or another beverage, preferably with meals to enhance absorption and minimize gastrointestinal upset. Some supplements may recommend a specific dosing schedule or additional dietary and lifestyle recommendations to support overall health and well-being.

Side Effects: Spirulina supplements are generally well-tolerated by most people when used as directed, but some individuals may experience side effects such as gastrointestinal upset, allergic reactions, or interactions with medications. It's essential to read the ingredient list carefully and avoid supplements containing ingredients that may trigger allergic reactions or interact with medications you're taking. Pregnant or breastfeeding women, individuals with certain medical conditions, or those taking medications should consult with a healthcare provider before using spirulina supplements. Additionally, it's important to choose supplements from reputable brands with third-party testing and certifications to ensure product quality and purity.

Steam Baths:

Definition: Steam baths, also known as steam rooms or steam saunas, are enclosed spaces where hot, humid air is generated by boiling water and released into the room. Steam baths are used for relaxation, detoxification, and promoting overall health and well-being.

Ingredients: Steam baths require water and a heat source, typically a steam generator or boiler, to produce steam. The steam itself is the active ingredient in steam baths, providing heat and humidity to the body.

How to Prepare: Preparing for a steam bath involves selecting a suitable steam room or facility and ensuring that it's properly heated and ventilated. It's essential to hydrate adequately before and after a steam bath to prevent dehydration and to listen to your body's cues to avoid overheating.

Dosage: The duration and frequency of steam bath sessions can vary depending on individual preferences and tolerance to heat. A typical steam bath session may last 10 to 20 minutes, although some people may prefer shorter or longer sessions.

How to Use: To use a steam bath, enter the steam room and sit or lie comfortably, allowing the hot, humid air to envelop your body. It's important to breathe deeply and relax during the session, allowing the steam to penetrate the skin and promote sweating and detoxification. After the designated time, exit the steam room, cool down gradually, and rehydrate with water or electrolyte-rich beverages.

Side Effects: Steam baths are generally safe for most people when used appropriately, but they can pose risks if not practiced correctly. Potential side effects of steam baths may include dehydration, heat exhaustion, heatstroke, dizziness, fainting, and exacerbation of certain medical conditions (such as cardiovascular disease or low blood pressure). It's important to stay hydrated, limit steam bath sessions to a safe duration, and avoid excessive heat exposure if pregnant, breastfeeding, or if you have certain health conditions. Individuals with underlying health concerns should consult with a healthcare provider before starting steam bath therapy to ensure it's safe and appropriate for them.

Sugar Detox:

Definition: A sugar detox is a dietary approach aimed at reducing or eliminating added sugars from the diet for a specified period.

It's designed to break dependence on sugar, reset taste buds, improve metabolic health, and reduce cravings for sweet foods.

Ingredients: A sugar detox involves eliminating or minimizing foods and beverages that contain added sugars, such as sugary snacks, desserts, sweetened beverages, processed foods, and condiments with added sugars. Instead, it emphasizes whole, unprocessed foods such as fruits, vegetables, lean proteins, whole grains, nuts, seeds, and healthy fats.

How to Prepare: Preparing for a sugar detox involves cleaning out your pantry and refrigerator of sugary foods and stocking up on nutritious, whole foods. It's essential to read food labels carefully to identify hidden sources of added sugars and to plan meals and snacks that are free from added sugars.

Dosage: The duration of a sugar detox can vary depending on individual goals and preferences. Some people may choose to do a short-term sugar detox lasting a few days to a week, while others may opt for a longer-term approach lasting several weeks or more. It's important to set realistic goals and listen to your body's cues during the detox process.

How to Use: During a sugar detox, focus on eating whole, nutrient-dense foods that are naturally low in sugar and high in fiber, protein, and healthy fats. This may include plenty of fruits and vegetables, lean proteins such as poultry, fish, tofu, and legumes, whole grains such as quinoa and brown rice, nuts and seeds, and healthy fats such as avocados and olive oil. Be mindful of your sugar intake from natural sources such as fruits and limit added sugars from processed foods and beverages.

Side Effects: A sugar detox may initially cause side effects such as cravings, mood swings, headaches, fatigue, and irritability as the body adjusts to lower sugar intake. These symptoms are usually temporary and subside with time. It's important to stay hydrated, eat balanced meals, and get plenty of sleep during the detox process to support overall well-being. If you have specific health concerns or medical conditions, consult with a healthcare provider or registered dietitian before starting a sugar detox to ensure it's safe and appropriate for you.

THE END